Eat to Live Diet For Beginners:

Fast and Healthy Weight Loss Program to Lose Body Fat, Get Flat Belly and Slim Body, Lower Blood Pressure

By

Brittany Samons

Table of Contents

Introduction 5

Chapter 1. Diet Principles 6

Chapter 2. Good Types of Foods to Eat For Losing Weight 10

Chapter 3. Foods to Take to Reduce High Blood Pressure . 17

Chapter 4. Foods to Be Avoided For High Blood Pressure.. 21

Chapter 5. Food Recipes For Good Diet Planning................ 25

    Food Recipe Examples 28

Final Words 30

Thank You Page.. 31

Eat to Live Diet For Beginners: Fast and Healthy Weight Loss Program to Lose Body Fat, Get Flat Belly and Slim Body, Lower Blood Pressure

By Brittany Samons

© Copyright 2015 Brittany Samons

Reproduction or translation of any part of this work beyond that permitted by section 107 or 108 of the 1976 United States Copyright Act without permission of the copyright owner is unlawful. Requests for permission or further information should be addressed to the author.

This publication is designed to provide accurate and authoritative information in regard to the subject matter covered. This work is sold with the understanding that the publisher is not engaged in rendering legal, accounting, or other professional services. If legal advice or other expert assistance is required, the services of a competent professional person should be sought.

First Published, 2015

Printed in the United States of America

Introduction

Living a healthy life is something that many people strive for. A healthy body always allows someone to appreciate and love him/herself. When we talk about maintaining your diet for good health, it doesn't mean that you should stick to one recipe plan. As much as you have a health body, it is good to take proper precautions to avoid unnecessary health problems. Take all kinds of foods but in a stipulated manner to avoid gaining weight. It is easy for anyone to watch out his/her eating habits. When you are told to take all kinds of food, consider moderating it and just eat some amount that fits your body. Avoid eating too much.

Chapter 1. Diet Principles

Here are some Eat to Live Diet principles to watch out.

1. **Do exercises**

Exercises are very important in our bodies. Person who does not engage his/her body for normal exercises can measly develop problems such as obesity or diseases such as diabetes. It is advisable to always do some exercises to your bodies. If you are a beginner, start by working every morning for 30 to 40 minutes. It will help a lot by burning those fats formed in your body. Ensure also to go to the gym and do all sorts of exercises there. It will really help you develop a healthy and stunning body.

2. **Eat all types of meals but appropriately**

Always make fruits and vegetables as part of your meal. Ensure those vegetables are rich in fiber. You can take the fruits an hour after you take your meals. You can add some meat like chicken or fish or mutton, but ensure to consume in smaller quantities. Health professionals have regularly been advising people to take a heavy and nutritious breakfast .it will sustain you for a longer period and help avoid taking food stuff in between the stipulated time which is three meals a day. When it comes to fruit juice, ensure that you drink fresh ones. Fruits will provide enough nutrients to your body.

3. **Eat food in time**

Taking food at any time is unhealthy to our bodies. If it is three meals a day ensure that you eat each one of them at the right time. It is very important as the brain as been set that at a certain time you have to eat. In case you take a meal at odd hours there will be an increased energy in your body. So ensure that you maintain the time you take food in each and every day.

4. **Avoid eating food in hurry**

Many of us work in offices or any other kind of jobs. Whenever we get some break for lunch we tend to take our food very fast. Health professionals advice that it is important for every person to take food within a period of around 20 minutes. That is the best time as the brain will decode information to your body. It will also ensure your stomach is not filled with a lot of food and the intestinal track. We normally tend to take a lot of food than what we should when we hurriedly eat. This is the most perfect way of adding unwanted weight to your body.

5. **Ensure to chew food**

It is good to chew every bit of your food before swallowing. You've got enough time to eat. Avoid hurrying. Remember that foods that are not properly chewed may lead to problems such as intestinal track blockage. Ensure also that you drink plenty of water. It is recommended that eight glasses of water each day is very health to our body. It helps in the process of burning those fats in our bodies.

6. **Do not skip breakfast**

Morning meals determine how your body will respond to other food stuff during the day. Taking breakfast is very important as your metabolism rate will be very high. In case you miss breakfast, your body will be very weak and not responsive. Taking many calories helps to burn during the day and release energy. Ensure that you take a lot of minerals and vitamins .You will always feel health and fit in your body.

Conclusion

Everyone can easily maintain a healthy diet. If you are that person who is very careful and loves living a health life ensure that you stick to these principles. They will really help you live young and always fit. You will always appreciate your body. Stay out of diseases and obesity. Don't ever dare skip some meals during the day just because you think skipping meals can help a lot. You will be creating more problems to your body weight. Also you can do regular exercises or visit a gym and do so there. You can also play with your kids while at home. This will help you a lot cut your weight and stay health for long. Be a watchdog of your body.

Chapter 2. Good Types of Foods to Eat For Losing Weight

Many people tend to think that taking a little amount of food is the best way for reducing body weight. But let me assure you that there some specific food kinds that one is always advised to take if the main agenda is to lose weight. Choosing the correct food for your diet is quit challenging and even frustrating. There are certain groups of food that play different roles in our bodies to improve our health. Here are some examples of food that can help burn fatty fats in your busy and ensure that you lose weight in a health way.

1. **Apple Cider Vinegar**

It is normally prepared by fermenting a apple cider. It contains a large amount of amino acids, vitamins enzymes and mineral salts. Health studies have proven that tasking a little amount of apple cider vinegar before any meal helps to increase the insulin sensitivity which will in turn ensure that insulin spikes is reduced which can end up cause cravings. Most foods include carbohydrates.

2. **Lemons**

It has also been proved that taking a glass of lemon water helps a lot cut your weight. Vitamin C. contained in it is able to oxidize 30 percent of more fats build up. It is always advisable to have high level of vitamin c in your body.

3. Grapefruits

This is type of fruits that contains low level of calories and high level of enzymes. Whenever you take it you will feel full for longer period of time. When taken every after meal, it will significantly reduce your body weight. It will also reduce formation of post glucose insulin levels.

4. Coconut oil

This is a powerful supplement that cuts your weight very fast. It is gaining much reputation due to its impressive abilities. They contain a medium chain fatty acids are normally used in the body for energy storage instead of fat breaking. The long chain fatty acids found in the body are burnt down to release the energy. Coconut oil one of the best in burning foods and fostering weight loss.

5. Pumpkin

This is the best food types for cutting your weight. The supplements found in pumpkin foster a great body loose as it will easily burn fats. It is one of the most delicious and health type of food.

6. **Eggs**

Though many people have a negative attitude towards eggs, it has been proven by health professionals as one of the best in reducing your weight. Eggs contain all kind of nutrients. It contains proteins which makes one full immediately which helps to gap food cravings. It also reduces the blood sugar; especially omelet. You can eventually increase your energy level and reduce cravings of food which will defiantly help eradicate gaining of weight. Instead you will be losing drastically.

7. **Salad**

Consuming high levels of salads before taking any heavy meal is good..Vegetables contain low level of calories and can easily fill your stomach instead of taking carbohydrates. Salads make good appetizers compared to other food stuffs that have been deeply fried or contain a high level of fats or calories. Salads of spinach, carrots, cabbage and potatoes can be the best.

8. Taking soups

Soups are very important in losing weight. Be it a chicken soup, fish or potatoes, whenever you take the soup it will suppress your appetite very fast. You can add maize beans or vegetables in your soup. It will enable the body to gain many vitamins which is very health.

9. Olive oil

Olive oils are very much healthier for consuming compared to butter and other fatty margarines e.g. blue band. It will speed up your metabolism rate, whereby fats will be broken to release energy for the body. It also solves health problems of the heart. It will also ensure that a lot of calories are burnt. With all this, your body will defiantly reduce 8iin a very systematic manner.

10. Cereals

Taking a lot of cereals especially in the morning will ensure that your body weight is reduced. Many of them contain a high level of fiber which helps in cutting weight. When a person takes food rich in fiber, it is always hard to feel an empty stomach. Avoid taking too much artificial cereals. They are not good for our bodies.

11. Celery

This type of vegetable that a cut down your weight by reducing appetites. It has very low in calories and contains a lot of fiber. Celery also has a good test and it is crunchy when consumed. It is one of the best foods that health professionals' advice people with a lot of body weight to take. You can eat as much as you want without gaining any weight.

12. Lentils

Lentils are a type of food which contains powerful minerals that can easily cut your weight. It also fosters the metabolism reaction in the body and also contains fiber in large quantity which makes one feel full for longer period of time. Their digestion process in the body is very slower, which makes one not to feel hungry very fast. Lentils are also advantageous as they can be cooked in different styles e.g. dip sauce soup or s side dishes in main foods.

13. Pickles

They are a type of snacks made from cucumber trees. They contain low level of calories which foster easy digestion and one can eat as much as he/she wants without adding any weight. They also act as immune to our bodies. They are found in different forms e, g salt, sour or baked. It is one of the best weight loss type of snack.

14. Meat

Many people fear taking meat due to the fact that it will defiantly increase body weight. You got it wrong, as long as you consider taking those that does not contain steroids and hormones you will never add any weight. Apparently, taking proteins fosters the reaction of metabolism rate which is well associated with weight loss in our bodies. Proteins helps one from overeating and keeps you full for long

Conclusion

Taking a healthy diet food wants someone who is really very serious. Always check the ingredients in your food and consider taking ones that contain the above ones. Don't take losing weight as something that will take you ages to achieve it. It only needs some devotion and hard work and all will be well.

Chapter 3. Foods to Take to Reduce High Blood Pressure

Hypertension has been one of the most threatening diseases currently in the world. It has wiped many faces both young and old from the world. There are several factors that can lead to high blood pressure. They include obesity, chronic stress genes of your family or smoking. Some of the causes can be easily prevented e.g. smoking. One can be advised to quit smoking to stay out of such dangers. When suffering from hypertension, there are some foods that you will likely have to take. This type of foods ensures that your blood level is well maintained at a certain speed all through. Here are some of the foods.

1. **Take Quinoa meals**

It is normally found in South Africa. The plant bears fruits. It contains fiber which helps remove all toxic materials in the arteries and reduce the level of sodium. It has been clinically proved as the best in reducing the speed of blood level in the body. The more you take the fiber the more the sodium and fats you can gain on daily basis.

2. Drink apple juice

Due to the high level f cholesterol formation, it is considered that taking apple juice on daily basis can have a great impact on the cardiac system. The apple juice help reduce the LDL oxidation which will in turn lower the speed of blood in arteries. It will also foster proper circulation of blood all over the body.

3. Take Saffron spice

This is a very special type of spice that can be added to meals the same way like ginger. It falls among the most considered foods for reducing hypertension. It plays a great role in lowering the blood speed in the arteries and other parts o09f the body.

4. Bananas

This is a type of fruit that is sometimes considered as stable food for some communities in the world. It can be either cooked or eaten when it ah ribbed. It contains potassium which is essential for lowering the blood pressure level. Health professionals have advised that is heal6th for someone suffering from high blood pressure to consume 3 bananas every day to help increase the potassium content in the body.

5. **Regular physical exercise**

Having regular physical exercise is very important for the body. When you do some exercises regularly, the heart and the vessels will function very well. Uncontrolled high blood pressure has generated many risks which include having a heart attack or stroke. When you see those people who normally do a lot of exercises, you will find that the heart rate is very normal and the blood pressure is low. Always engage yourself in physical activities. It will help you eradicate problems such as obesity which is a dangerous kind of body weight that can lead to hypertension.

6. **Consume low level of fats**

Ensure that the calories you consume are less than 30 percent made of fat. Always stay away from fatty foods. Take meat such as for chicken or fish as it contains very low level of calories.

Conclusion

It is always important to reduce your blood pressure. The more you reduce the more you get to prevent it and live a health life. Many people opt to medicine mostly and leave such foods which are very strong in reducing hypertension. If you really need to survive for a long period, ensure that you consume those food that can help you fight against high blood pressure. Do not be deceived that you can only take medication and be quite well. You can as well take care of your body. It does not a lot of efforts or sacrifices. And it will never cost you at all.

Chapter 4. Foods to Be Avoided For High Blood Pressure

High blood pressure is a very dangerous dieses .If it is left unchecked for long period it may lead to damage of the vascular and retinal changes. It is always important to consider pharmacological ways instead of relying on medical treatment only. Patients suffering from high blood pressure should suddenly avoid some foods which may trigger the pressure level of the blood. It is also advisable to regularly check your blood pressure to ensure that it is well maintained in such a way that it may not cause any problems in your daily life. When also suffering from hypertension, avoid having mind stress, stress can cost you a lot as the state of your mind is not relaxed which trigger high blood pressure in the body. Always can consider having peace of mind and avoid such problems. Here are some kinds of food that should be avoided.

1. **Salts**

Medical Researchers have found out that consuming a lot of dietary sodium is very dangerous to an hypertension patients. When large amount of sugar is taken, it is likely to trigger the rise of the blood pressure in your body. As time goes by the more salts you take the more the pressure advances each day. Salts have a restriction of consuming only about 100mmol per day. This level of consumption will ensure that the systolic blood pressure is reduced to a level of about of 8 to 14 mm Hg in several randomized placebo-controlled findings. In many cases, taking too many salts for a hypertension person might be much worst and can sometimes even lead to death.

When a lot of salt is consumed it will lead to more accumulation of fluids in the kidneys. With this case lot of pressure will be loaded in the heart which mill result to high level of blood pressure. If you are an hypertension patient, it is advisable to consume little amount of salt in each day. It will help you a lot as the less slats you take the high the reduction rate of your blood pressure in the body. Avoid food stuffs such as pizza, canned food, and salads. They contain high level of sodium which the body does not need. If you don't like taking much vegetables, white meat can be better e.g. fish chicken rather than the red meat. Avoid it in your diet all times to stay healthy always.

2. **Fats**

All kind of foods which contain a lot of fats should be avoided. Fats are very good in triggering the blood pressure in the body..Avoid foods such as, fatty meat, fried food, cream ice, cakes most snacks, cheese. Also avoid taking large consumption of foods containing fats and oils such as margarine for cooking vegetables, butter, fat back etc. When the density of lipoprotein is very low it will cause the thickening of the blood vessels which will cause extra pressure to be used to ensure blood flow in the body. Saturated fats are considered much worst for the heart and the blood vessels. Always take a diet that contains moderate fats or tans-fats.

3. **Caffeine intake**

The more the consumption of caffeine the body the more the blood pressure is increased in the body. Avoid regular coffee drinking habits. The consumption of 250mg of caffeine in the body on daily basis will eventually increase the systolic pressure from the normal 6mm Hg to 10mm Hg. This may cause a lot of problems in the blood pressure especially for hypertension patients.

4. **Alcohol consumption**

Alcohol as been one of the major causes of hypertension. When patients suffering from hypertension consume a lot of alcohol, it will raise their blood pressure when the level is reduced, the blood pressure level also drops down. Many patients suffering from hypertension are always advised to abstain from alcohol at all costs.

Conclusion

Hypertension patients can stay away from more sufferings if only they avoid taking large consumption of this food stuffs. High blood pressure can really damage your heart and blood vessels which can lead to early deaths. It is good to take those diets that your body can tolerate with. Always learn to appreciate who are no matter what challenges you are going through. Hypertension is a kind of diseases that can be easily controlled as long as you stay away from the above food stuffs.

Chapter 5. Food Recipes For Good Diet Planning

Eating a healthy diet is something that runs in every persons mind. You can take all kinds of food to ensure that your diet planning is maintained. But it is also good sometimes to watch out what kind of food should be taken at which time to avoid adding unwanted weight in your body. Having detox recipes is one of the most appropriate means of planning your daily diet. Taking a lot of fiber and drinking plenty of water is the most appropriate d way of maintain your health. Consuming a lot of vegetables, fruits beans and cereals is s good for your health. There are some kind of food recipes that one can easily take and feel well all through. These foods include:

1. **Alkaline raw soup**

Alkaline raw soup is very important to your diet. It will burn all the kinds of fats in the body. It is always made of onions, cucumber, avocado, s spinach garlic and red pepper. All this kind food materials play major roles in the body.

2. **Mediterranean diets**

This is very important diet that is gaining its popularity due its low level of fats. Mediterranean diets ensure that the body does not consume a lot of fats which can lead to gaining of weight. This type of food recipe is found online with body planning diet. It the most excellent type of recipe that every person should wish to take.

3. **Detox drinks**

This is a type of a detox that is made of fruit juice. The juice acts as cleaning method in the body, by removing all toxins around the body. Fresh juices are added in organic vegetables squeezed juice. You will defiantly come up with one of the best treatment for removing toxins and ensure that your body stays health.

4. **Gazpacho Soup**

This is a vegetable soup that is made by mixing garlic, bell peppers cucumber, tomatoes and bread that has been moistened and blended with olive oil, ice water and vinegar. It is always served while it is very cold. It is very good for planning your diet as it will ensure that it cleans the blood to ensure no pathogens are found in it. It initially originated from Spain but it currently used all over the world by many people who love maintaining their diets.

Food Recipe Examples

Breakfast Recipe

2 eggs mixed with spinach,1 teaspoon of butter or olive oil

1 slice of brown bread or organic turkey made sausage

Blueberries of ¼ cup or 1 celery mixed with almond water

In this type of breakfast, you will find that the food recipes are mostly oxidizers. They contain fewer fats and contain high level of grain products. This shows that the food will be burnt very slowly in the body, which will in turn release enough energy during the day.

Lunch recipe

4 roasted chicken breast, butter and garlic

Sea salt 1 teaspoon of butter and 1 cup of steamed carrots or roasted chicken with little amount of butter or garlic

½ a cup of rice mostly brown rice

In this recipe example you still find that there is very low consumption of fats. It contains a lot of proteins and fewer fats which is very suitable for the body.

Dinner recipe

Oz flounder containing little amount of garlic and butter

Sweet potato with three table spoon of butter

Swiss chard containing butter olive oil and almond

Again we find that in this recipe plan there is a very low oxidation due to the sweat potatoes and caneberries. This clearly indicates that, the oxidation rate should always come from a high level which is in the morning and end with low oxidizers at the end of the day.

Final Words

If any person sticks to such a meal plan, it will be very easy for him/her to maintain a good body weight and live a healthy diet. The real this is that matching your body with the correct diet that best suits your body will lead to health living. When preparing those meals, ensure that the supplements are well measured to foster your diet plan. This kind of recipe food shows how detoxification should happen during the day. When it is well followed, you will eventually lose some weight and have a great body fit which you will be well contended with it. The rule should always be avoiding consuming food stuffs that have been added something on top or sometimes extracted from it. Always consider taking natural food stuffs as they are considered the healthiest kinds of food.

Thank You Page

I want to personally thank you for reading my book. I hope you found information in this book useful and I would be very grateful if you could leave your honest review about this book. I certainly want to thank you in advance for doing this.

If you have the time, you can check my other books too.

www.ingramcontent.com/pod-product-compliance
Lightning Source LLC
LaVergne TN
LVHW021746060526
838200LV00052B/3509